Patients With Head Injury

Step by step Guide to Manage Head Injury Patient, Symptoms, First Aid, Treatment and Management Guidelines

Dan Phillips PhD

~DEDICATION~

~LARRY~

For your unwavering support, encouragement, and friendship. Your presence in my life has been a constant source of inspiration. Thank you for your invaluable kindness and belief in my journey. This book is a token of appreciation for your enduring friendship and steadfast encouragement.

TABLE OF CONTENT

CHAPTER 1. UNDERSTANDING HEAD INJURIES: ANATOMY AND MECHANISMS

This chapter could provide an overview of the different types of head injuries, their causes, and the anatomy of the head and brain. It sets the foundation for the reader's understanding of the topic.

CHAPTER 2. RECOGNIZING SYMPTOMS OF HEAD INJURY

This chapter would delve into the various symptoms that can arise after a head injury, including both immediate and delayed signs. It would help readers understand how to identify potential head injuries in patients.

CHAPTER 3. PROVIDING IMMEDIATE FIRST AID FOR HEAD INJURIES

In this chapter, you could outline the essential first aid measures that should be taken immediately after a head injury occurs. This might include steps like assessing consciousness, controlling bleeding, and stabilizing the patient.

Chapter 4. Diagnostic Procedures for Head Injury Patients

Here, you could explain the diagnostic methods used to assess the severity of head injuries, including imaging techniques like CT scans and MRI scans. It would provide insight into how medical professionals determine the extent of the injury.

Chapter 5. Treatment Approaches for Head Injury Patients

This chapter would explore the various treatment options available for head injury patients, ranging from conservative management to surgical interventions. It could cover topics like medication, monitoring, and the decision-making process for surgical cases.

CHAPTER 6. NEUROLOGICAL MANAGEMENT AND REHABILITATION

DISCUSS THE SPECIALIZED CARE REQUIRED FOR PATIENTS WITH NEUROLOGICAL DEFICITS RESULTING FROM HEAD INJURIES. COVER TOPICS LIKE NEUROREHABILITATION, PHYSICAL THERAPY, OCCUPATIONAL THERAPY, AND SPEECH THERAPY.

CHAPTER 7. PSYCHOLOGICAL AND EMOTIONAL SUPPORT FOR PATIENTS AND FAMILIES

ADDRESS THE EMOTIONAL AND PSYCHOLOGICAL ASPECTS OF HEAD INJURIES, BOTH FOR PATIENTS AND THEIR FAMILIES. THIS COULD INCLUDE COPING STRATEGIES, SUPPORT GROUPS, AND WAYS TO NAVIGATE THE EMOTIONAL CHALLENGES THAT ARISE DURING RECOVERY.

CHAPTER 8. LONG-TERM MANAGEMENT AND PREVENTION STRATEGIES

THIS CHAPTER WOULD FOCUS ON THE ONGOING MANAGEMENT OF HEAD INJURY PATIENTS, INCLUDING LONG-TERM MEDICAL FOLLOW-UP, POTENTIAL COMPLICATIONS, AND STRATEGIES TO

PREVENT FUTURE HEAD INJURIES. IT MIGHT ALSO
TOUCH ON LIFESTYLE ADJUSTMENTS AND SAFETY
MEASURES.

CHAPTER 1

Understanding Head Injuries: Anatomy and Mechanisms

Head injuries are a complicated and dangerous medical condition that can arise from a variety of situations, including falls, accidents, sports-related mishaps, and more. We will explore the complex world of head injuries in this introductory chapter, illuminating their different forms, underlying causes, and the key anatomical components in the head and brain that are affected. Readers will be better prepared to understand the following chapters, which concentrate on managing and treating patients afflicted by head injuries, if they have a thorough understanding of the complex aspects of brain injuries and their mechanisms.

Head and Brain Anatomy: An Intricate Network of Structures

Encompassing a multitude of essential organs, sensory systems, and the most complex structure of all, the brain, the human skull is a marvel of natural design. One must first become familiar with the various parts of the cranium in order to comprehend head injuries. The skull serves as both the structural support for the face and a hard shell that encloses and protects the brain. A complex system of cerebral spinal fluid channels, cranial nerves, and blood arteries runs beneath the surface of the skull, cooperating to preserve the delicate balance required for normal brain function.

Different cognitive, sensory, and motor functions are attributed to different regions of the brain. With its noticeable creases and fissures, the cerebrum governs conscious thought, willpower, and voluntary motions.

The brainstem controls essential processes including breathing, heart rate, and consciousness, whereas the cerebellum coordinates balance, coordination, and fine motor control. The understanding of how brain traumas can have a wide range of repercussions on an individual's physical and cognitive well-being is based on this complex network of interrelated regions.

Head Injury Mechanisms: Deciphering the Causes

Numerous methods can result in head injuries, and each has the potential to have negative effects of its own. Gaining an appreciation of these mechanisms is essential to comprehending the variety of brain injuries and how they affect patients.

Injury by Blunt Force: When the head is struck by an outside object, the skull absorbs the impact, which may lead to fractures or contusions. Physical assaults, car crashes, and falls are frequently the cause of blunt force injuries.

- Injuries with penetration: Depending on the site of entry, sharp items that pierce the skull, like bullets or sharp tools, can cause localized injury to particular parts of the brain.

- Whiplash: An Acceleration-Deceleration Injury The brain may migrate inside the skull as a result of abrupt, violent head movements. This movement may result in diffuse axonal damage, shearing stresses, and the stretching or ripping of sensitive neuronal connections.

Crystal Trauma: Even in the absence of a direct hit, explosions can produce shockwaves that have an influence on the brain. Rapid pressure fluctuations have the potential to cause harm from secondary debris as well as the main shockwave.

- Spinal Traumas: Brain damage can result from a head that rotates or twists quickly. The rotational forces involved in these injuries frequently result in diffuse damage across several regions of the brain.

Various Head Injury Types: A Range of Severity

From minor concussions to potentially fatal traumatic brain injuries, head traumas can range widely in severity. Comprehending these categorizations facilitates assessing the possible influence on patients.

A minor traumatic brain injury caused by a sudden hit to the head or jolt is known as a concussion. Concussions usually go away with time, though they might cause transient cognitive and physical deficits.

- Verdict: a localized bruise brought on by blunt force injuries to the surface of the brain. Neurological problems may result from a contusion, depending on its size and location.

A fracture of the skull, a break in one of the cranial bones. Broken bones can be either depressed or linear, and depending on the severity of the blow, they may or may not cause brain damage.

- Axonal Diffuse Injury: This injury involves disruption to the neuronal connections in the brain and is brought on by rotating or shearing pressures. Widespread cognitive and functional problems may ensue from it.

- Hematoma: Blood clot caused by broken blood arteries that accumulates inside the brain. If hematomas are not treated right away, they may put pressure on brain tissue and result in serious harm.

To sum up, this chapter provides an essential basis for understanding the complexities of head injuries. It will be easier for readers to traverse the next chapters that discuss the management, treatment, and care of patients impacted by these injuries if they have a solid understanding of the anatomy of the head and brain as well as the various mechanisms and types of injuries that can occur. Having a firm grasp of the fundamentals will enable caregivers, patients, and healthcare providers to make wise decisions and help those affected by head injuries recover.

CHAPTER 2

Recognizing Symptoms of Head Injury

A head injury is a severe medical condition that can affect a person's health and well-being both immediately and over time. It's critical to recognize the signs of a brain injury, regardless of the cause—accidents, falls, sports-related mishaps, or other traumatic events. In-depth discussion of both immediate and delayed symptoms following a head injury is provided in Chapter 2, which also gives readers the knowledge they need to recognize possible head injuries in patients.

Comprehending the Intricacy of Brain Traumas:

Understand the intricacy of head traumas before diving into the symptoms. Almost every part of our bodies is controlled by the delicate and complex brain. The structures and functions of the brain can be affected by trauma, which can result in a variety of symptoms that might not show up right away. Early diagnosis and recognition of these symptoms can have a substantial impact on the course of treatment and recovery.

Short-Term Symptoms:

1. Consciousness Loss (LOC): Loss of consciousness is one of the easiest indicators of a serious head injury to recognize. Even though loss of consciousness can occur for short or long periods of time, all cases of LOC need to be treated medically right once.

2. Bewilderment and Disorientation: After suffering a brain injury, people may become disoriented, confused, and have trouble focusing. They can struggle to remember what happened before the accident or might not be able to identify familiar faces or locations.

3. Vomiting and Nausea: After a head injury, abnormalities in the brain's normal functioning may give rise to these symptoms. Severe or prolonged nausea and vomiting need to be treated seriously.

4. Brain: Severe and ongoing headaches, particularly ones that get

worse over time, may be an indication of a serious brain injury. Light and sound sensitivities might accompany headaches.

5. Inequitable Students or Shifts in Vision: A brain injury affecting the nerves and structures responsible for vision can be indicated by dilated or uneven pupils, blurred vision, or other alterations in vision.

Postponed Symptoms:

1. Variations in Mood and Personality: After suffering a brain injury, people may exhibit mood swings, irritability, or personality

changes for several days or weeks. Anxiety and depression could also emerge.

2. Cognitive Impairments: In the days or weeks after a head injury, memory issues, concentration issues, and less mental clarity may become noticeable. The way a person lives and functions on a daily basis may be impacted by these cognitive deficits.

3. Sleep disruptions: Following a head injury, insomnia, excessive sleep, or other sleep disruptions may occur. Sleep disturbances might also make the healing process more difficult.

Sensory Changes: Modifications in sensory perception, ringing in the ears (tinnitus), or loss of taste or smell may be signs of underlying brain injury.

5. Seizures: It's important to pay attention to seizures that happen days, weeks, or even months after a head injury. They might be a sign of persistent brain disorders.

When Medical Help Is Needed:

When it comes to brain injuries, it is crucial to get medical help as soon as possible. Since symptoms are frequently not immediately apparent, alertness and vigilance are essential. If you or someone you know goes through any of the following, you need to get medical attention immediately:

Becoming unconscious, even for a little while
Heaps that are persistent or getting worse
- Weakness or numbness in limbs - Confusion, confusion, or difficulty speaking - Seizures
- Frequent nausea or vomiting - Vision abnormalities, such as dilated pupils or uneven pupils - Emotional or personality swings - Sleep difficulties

- The discharge of clear liquid or blood from the nose or ears

Rendering:

The significance of identifying brain injury symptoms is emphasized in Chapter 2 in order to guarantee prompt medical attention. Both immediate and delayed symptoms provide important information about the seriousness and possible aftereffects of a brain injury. Whether it's a small bump or a serious knock to the head, knowing the spectrum of symptoms can enable people to take the necessary precautions for their own or their loved ones' health. This chapter provides readers with important information on the intricacies of brain injuries and the range of symptoms that may appear. It also helps readers recognize and treat head injuries carefully and diligently.

CHAPTER 3

Providing Immediate First Aid for Head Injuries

In this chapter, you could outline the essential first aid measures that should be taken immediately after a head injury occurs. This might include steps like assessing consciousness, controlling bleeding, and stabilizing the patient.

Provided quickly and appropriately in the critical moments after a head injury, first aid can significantly impact the patient's prognosis. The purpose of this chapter is to provide readers with the information and abilities needed to provide patients with head injuries with prompt and efficient first aid. Anyone who might find themselves in a situation where they need immediate assistance should be aware of the processes listed here, from determining the extent of the damage to taking precautions against future issues.

Consciousness Assessment: Glasgow Coma Scale

Using the Glasgow Coma Scale (GCS), one of the first steps in administering first aid for a head injury is determining the patient's degree of consciousness. Three elements are assessed by this scale: verbal reaction, physical response, and eye-opening response. The total score directs further steps and aids in assessing the severity of the brain injury. A lower GCS score indicates a more serious injury and the requirement for immediate medical care.

Managing Bleeding and Reducing Additional Damage

Head injuries frequently cause bleeding, which can be internal (found inside the skull) or external (visible). When dealing with external bleeding, the flow should be controlled by gently pressing with a clean cloth or bandage. It is imperative to refrain from applying undue pressure since this may worsen the damage.

It's critical to identify symptoms of internal bleeding, such as altered behavior, disorientation, slurred speech, or a growing headache. Neurological symptoms that worsen quickly may be a sign of increasing intracranial pressure brought on by bleeding. It is crucial to keep the patient motionless and to refrain from any actions that can cause the blood flow to the head to rise.

Keeping the Patient Stabilized: The ABCs

It is crucial to make sure the patient's breathing, circulation, and airway—or the ABCs—are stable. The recovery position helps keep the patient's airway open and lowers the chance that they will choke on saliva or vomit if they are unconscious. The patient should receive cardiopulmonary resuscitation (CPR) as soon as possible if they are not breathing.

Retaining adequate circulation is essential to avoid shock, which is made worse by head trauma. It is crucial to start basic life support measures while waiting for medical assistance if the patient's condition worsens.

Keeping an Eye on Vital Signs and Dialing for Medical Assistance

critical indicators such as blood pressure, heart rate, and breathing rate should be continuously monitored since they provide critical information about the health of the patient. Any abrupt changes could be a sign of other problems or increased intracranial pressure.

It's critical to get emergency medical assistance if you have moderate to severe head injuries. Medical personnel possess the knowledge and resources necessary to conduct a thorough assessment of the injury and make well-informed judgments about the course of treatment and transfer to a medical facility.

Reducing Motion and Assisting the Affected Person

Minimize the wounded person's mobility as soon as the emergency first aid measures are in place to avoid aggravating the injury. If necessary, immobilizing the head and neck can assist avert any spinal cord injury. Furthermore, reducing tension and anxiety during this crucial period can be achieved by providing consolation and assurance to the patient and those nearby.

To sum up, this chapter provides guidance on the critical first aid actions that need to be performed right away in the event of a brain injury. Through comprehension of the importance of determining consciousness, managing bleeding, stabilizing the patient, keeping an eye on vital signs, and obtaining expert medical assistance, readers will be more prepared to act with efficiency in emergency scenarios. When it comes to brain injury patients' overall prognosis and recuperation, prompt and adequate first aid can make a big difference.

CHAPTER 4

Diagnostic Procedures for Head Injury Patients

Here, you could explain the diagnostic methods used to assess the severity of head injuries, including imaging techniques like CT scans and MRI scans. It would provide insight into how medical professionals determine the extent of the injury.

A prompt and precise diagnosis is crucial for assessing the severity of head injuries and directing the most suitable course of therapy. In-depth discussion of the complex realm of diagnostic techniques used by doctors to evaluate head injuries is provided in Chapter 3. This chapter provides information on how medical professionals determine the extent of a brain injury, facilitating well-informed decision-making and the best possible patient care. Methods range from conventional physical examinations to cutting-edge imaging techniques like CT and MRI scans.

The Value of a Precise Diagnosis:

There is a large range of severity when it comes to head injuries, from minor concussions to serious traumatic brain injuries (TBIs). In addition to helping medical personnel analyze the immediate damage, the diagnostic process also helps them plan for the patient's long-term rehabilitation and foresee prospective difficulties. A thorough understanding of diagnostic techniques enables medical professionals to give individualized treatment and interventions catered to each patient's particular requirements.

Physical Assessment:

The first step in assessing a patient who has had a brain injury is frequently a comprehensive physical examination. Health care providers evaluate neurological function, vital signs, and cognitive state. Important elements of the assessment consist of:

The Glasgow Coma Scale (GCS) is as follows: This standardized test assesses the verbal, motor, and visual responses of the patient. The GCS score helps categorize the severity of a brain injury and offers a measurable indicator of awareness.

2. Neurological Assessment: Health care providers assess reflexes, coordination, and sensory and motor function. Any abnormalities or deficiencies may point to certain brain regions that are involved.

Image-Using Methods:

Modern imaging techniques are essential for identifying and classifying head injuries. By using these approaches, medical experts can evaluate the level of damage by seeing precise visualizations of the brain's components. The following are the two main imaging modalities used to diagnose head injuries:

1. CT (Computerized Tomography) Scan: CT scans produce cross-sectional images of the brain using X-rays. When it comes to spotting fractures, acute bleeding, and other structural irregularities, they are especially helpful. Because CT scans are quick and accessible, they are an essential tool in emergency situations.

2. MRI Scan: Magnetic Resonance Imaging MRI scans create finely detailed images of the soft tissues in the brain by using radio waves and

strong magnets. When it comes to identifying minor injuries like contusions and diffuse axonal injuries, MRIs are quite helpful. They could take longer to complete, but they offer a more thorough understanding of brain architecture and pathophysiology.

Extra Diagnostic Resources:

In some circumstances, medical practitioners may use extra diagnostic instruments to obtain thorough data regarding the brain injury:

1. Monitoring Intracranial Pressure (ICP): A probe is inserted into the

skull during this intrusive operation to assess the pressure inside the brain. Treatment choices may be influenced by elevated ICP, which can reveal edema or hemorrhage.

2. A EEG (Electroencephalogram): EEG captures brain electrical activity and can be used to detect abnormalities, such seizures, that may not be visible with conventional diagnostic techniques.

3. Neurovascular Angiography: In order to see blood flow within the brain, contrast dye is injected into blood vessels during this operation. It

is helpful in evaluating vascular anomalies and damage.

Examining and Applying Diagnostic Results:

Treatment planning and management are based on the data acquired from diagnostic tests. Medical practitioners evaluate the results to assess the extent of the damage, anticipate future issues, and customize treatments to the patient's requirements. Additionally, the diagnostic procedure helps with tracking the patient's development over time and modifying treatment plans as needed.

Interdisciplinary Method:

Collaboration between different medical specialties, such as neurologists, neurosurgeons, radiologists, and critical care physicians, is frequently necessary for the diagnosis and treatment of head injuries. By using a multidisciplinary approach, the patient is guaranteed to receive all-encompassing care that takes into account the short- and long-term effects of the injury.

Rendering:

A thorough description of the diagnostic techniques used by doctors to evaluate head injuries is provided in Chapter 3. Advanced imaging techniques such as CT and MRI scans, as well as physical tests that assess brain function, are essential diagnostic tools that help determine the degree of damage and direct therapy choices. This chapter gives readers a better understanding of how medical professionals assess head injuries by exploring the complexities of diagnostic techniques. This helps readers recognize how difficult it can be to diagnose head injuries and how crucial accurate assessment is to achieving the best possible outcomes for patients.

CHAPTER 5

Treatment Approaches for Head Injury Patients

This chapter would explore the various treatment options available for head injury patients, ranging from conservative management to surgical interventions. It could cover topics like medication, monitoring, and the decision-making process for surgical cases.

To achieve the best results when treating patients with brain injuries, a thorough and knowledgeable approach is necessary. This chapter explores the range of potential treatment options, which include conservative care and surgical treatments. Caretakers and medical professionals can make decisions that best promote patient recovery by being aware of the various strategies discussed in this chapter. These strategies range from symptom-relieving medications to careful monitoring and the complex decision-making process around surgeries.

Economic Stewardship:

Conservative management is the use of non-invasive techniques, mainly supportive care and close observation, to treat head injuries. In cases of mild concussions and small brain injuries, this might be the main treatment plan. Among the essential elements of conservative management are:

Relaxation and Thoughts: It's important to give the brain enough time to recuperate. Rest—both mental and physical—is advised. It is imperative to closely observe any alterations in neurological status or symptoms.

Pain Management: Over-the-Counter analgesics can make headaches and other discomforts go away. But care should be taken to steer clear of drugs that can thin the blood and raise the chance of bleeding.

Symptom Handling: It's critical to treat particular symptoms like nausea, vertigo, or sleep difficulties in order to ensure patient comfort. Both lifestyle modifications and anti-nausea drugs may be helpful.

Pharmaceuticals:

To treat both the physical and cognitive components of a head injury, different drugs may be used, depending on the severity and particular symptoms:

Pain Relievers: Over-the-counter analgesics such as acetaminophen are effective in treating headaches and pain.

Anti-Inflammatory medications: NSAIDs, or non-steroidal anti-inflammatory medications, have the ability to lessen inflammation and discomfort.

- Medications to Prevent Epilepsy: Patients who have had head injuries and are at risk of seizures may be offered anti-epileptic drugs.

Medications for Sedatives or Anti-Anxiety: These may be taken into account if the patient has trouble falling asleep, is anxious, or is restless.

Observation and Monitoring:

No matter whether strategy is selected, individuals with brain injuries require close care. Frequent neurological examinations, which include evaluations of speech, motor abilities, cognitive function, and pupil reactions, offer valuable information about the patient's development. Any worsening of the neurological condition or symptoms should be treated with medical attention very once.

Medical Procedures:

Surgical treatments may be required in cases of moderate to severe head injuries in order to relieve pressure on the brain or repair physical damage. Surgical techniques consist of:

- Hysterectomy: a kind of surgery when a portion of the skull is removed in order to access and treat brain injury.

Hematoma Removal: In order to release pressure on the brain, surgical evacuation may be required if there is an accumulation of blood inside the skull.

Discompressive Head Extraction: It may be necessary to temporarily remove a part of the skull in order to allow the brain to enlarge without compression if intracranial pressure rises to dangerously high levels.

Process of Making Decisions:

The kind and extent of the brain injury, the patient's general health, and the way they respond to early therapies all play a role in determining the best course of treatment. To decide on the best course of action, medical experts consult with neurologists, neurosurgeons, and other specialists.

This chapter concludes with a thorough summary of the various treatment modalities accessible to individuals with brain injuries. Every approach, from conservative care to surgical interventions, is customized based on the individual patient's needs and the extent of the injury. Knowing these options gives patients, caregivers, and healthcare professionals the information they need to make decisions that promote the best possible outcome and enhanced quality of life.

CHAPTER 6

Neurological Management and
Rehabilitation

Discuss the specialized care required for patients with neurological deficits resulting from head injuries. Cover topics like neurorehabilitation, physical therapy, occupational therapy, and speech therapy.

Brain injury-related neurological impairments can significantly affect a person's functional independence and quality of life. The comprehensive rehabilitation procedures and specialized treatment needed to address these deficiencies are covered in detail in Chapter 6. This chapter discusses the multidisciplinary strategy required for treating patients with head injuries in order to promote recovery, restore function, and improve their overall well-being. This approach includes physical therapy, occupational therapy, speech therapy, and neurorehabilitation.

Knowing What Neurological Deficits Are:

Numerous neurological problems, such as motor impairments, cognitive issues, and communication difficulties, can result from head injuries. The degree and location of the brain injury determine the kind and severity of these deficits. In order to reduce long-term deficits and increase recovery potential, comprehensive neurological treatment and rehabilitation are crucial.

Rehabilitation for neurons:

Treating neurological impairments with a thorough and individualized approach is called neurorehabilitation. It entails a blend of therapeutic, medical, and behavioral interventions with the goal of fostering functional improvement, adaptive strategies, and neuronal healing. Important elements of neurorehabilitation consist of:

1. Physical Therapy: To enhance strength, balance, coordination, and mobility, physical therapists create customized exercise regimens. They collaborate closely with patients to improve their physical functioning and regained motor abilities.

2.   Occupational   Therapy: Occupational therapists work to improve and restore a person's capacity to carry out everyday tasks like getting dressed, taking care of themselves, and preparing meals. They support patients in creating plans to maximize their independence and adjusting to functional limits.

3. Speech Pathology: Communication deficiencies, such as issues with speech, language comprehension, and cognitive-communication abilities, are addressed by speech-language pathologists. They offer methods for enhancing swallowing and speaking skills.

4. Cognitive Rehabilitation: Following head injuries, cognitive deficiencies, such as memory and attention problems, are frequently observed. Programs for cognitive rehabilitation use strategies to strengthen cognitive abilities, encourage problem-solving, and enhance general cognitive function.

Interprofessional Cooperation:

Neurologists, physiatrists, psychologists, nurses, and therapists are just a few of the healthcare specialists who must work together successfully to manage and rehabilitate neurological conditions. Together, the members of this interdisciplinary team create a thorough treatment plan that is customized to the needs and objectives of each patient.

Assigning Reasonable Objectives:
Since neurological healing is a long process, it is essential to create reasonable goals in order to keep patients motivated and involved. Rehabilitation specialists collaborate closely with patients and their families to set realistic goals, monitor development, and modify the treatment plan as necessary.

Technological Innovation:

The subject of neurological rehabilitation has changed as a result of technological advancements. Modern tools like virtual reality and robotically assisted therapy provide patients dynamic, entertaining environments in which to hone their motor and cognitive abilities. These tools promote active engagement and improve the recovery process.

Psychosocial and Emotional Assistance:

Patients and their families may experience emotional and

psychosocial effects from head trauma. Psychological support is a component of rehabilitation programs that helps with problems including anxiety, depression, and adjusting to the difficulties caused by neurological limitations. Counseling and support groups give people a forum to talk about their experiences and coping mechanisms.

Emergency Medical Care and Aftercare:

Neurological rehabilitation can last for months or even years; it is not limited to a set amount of time. Frequent follow-up evaluations enable medical staff to keep an eye on the patient's progress, make any required corrections, and offer continuing support as they work toward recovery.

Rendering:

In Chapter 6, the significance of neurological care and rehabilitation is emphasized as a means of tackling the complex issues associated with head trauma. The goal of the multidisciplinary approach is to improve the entire quality of life for individuals with neurological abnormalities by enhancing recovery, restoring function, and providing emotional support in addition to physical therapy and cognitive training. This chapter helps readers comprehend the importance of specialist treatment and rehabilitation following brain injuries by shedding light on these all-encompassing tactics. This helps readers gain a deeper comprehension of the process leading to recovery and restoration.

CHAPTER 7

Psychological and Emotional Support for Patients and Families

Address the emotional and psychological aspects of head injuries, both for patients and their families. This could include coping strategies, support groups, and ways to navigate the emotional challenges that arise during recovery.

Head injuries have a significant psychological and emotional impact on victims as well as their relatives, in addition to their physical effects. This chapter explores the sometimes disregarded psychological side of recovery: the emotional path that goes hand in hand with the physical healing process. Through discussing the psychological aspects, providing coping mechanisms, and outlining available resources, this chapter seeks to provide patients, caregivers, and families with the necessary tools to successfully negotiate the complex emotional terrain of the recovery process.

Aware of the Emotional Effects:

Many emotional reactions, such as worry, despair, annoyance, and even personality changes, can result from a head injury. These emotional shifts could be from the actual injury, changes in brain chemistry, or difficulties adjusting to a new environment.

Coping Techniqucs:

Giving patients useful coping mechanisms can help them deal with the psychological effects of a head injury:

Psychotherapy: Patients can regulate their anxiety, address mood swings, and create good coping mechanisms with the aid of cognitive behavioral therapy (CBT) and other psychotherapies.

Relaxation and Mindfulness Methods: Relaxation techniques and mindfulness meditation help lower stress, strengthen emotional control, and boost general wellbeing.

- Reporting: Encouragement of journaling as a means of expressing ideas and feelings might give patients a way to manage their emotions and monitor their progress.

Social Support: Encouraging patients to draw from their support system, which includes friends, family, and support groups, can help them feel less alone and more like they belong.

Helping Families:

A head injury affects not just the victim but also their family. It's critical to provide emotional support and direction:

- Schooling: Helping families better comprehend and deal with the difficulties might be achieved by educating them about the possible psychological changes that may take place.

- Open Communication: Promoting candid discussions about feelings, anxieties, and worries within the family can help to strengthen harmony and understanding.

Counseling Services for Families: Families can learn how to best support their loved one's rehabilitation and deal with the changes they're going through by having access to therapy or support groups.

Managing Emotional Difficulties:

Recovery's emotional journey isn't straight line and might have highs and lows:

- Celebrating Small Victories: No matter how tiny a victory may be, it can still raise spirits and give a feeling of accomplishment.

- Addressing Frustrations: Promoting open communication between patients and providers about frustrations and limitations can help shield them from feelings of powerlessness and loneliness.

Achieving Reasonable Expectations: Setting realistic expectations and goals with patients and their families can help them feel accomplished and avoid disappointment.

Resources and Support Groups:

Patients and their families can share stories, get advice from others who have been there before, and find comfort in the company of like-minded individuals in support groups. Local support groups, forums, and online tools can all offer priceless connections and a feeling of belonging.

This chapter concludes by emphasizing how critical it is to understand the psychological and emotional difficulties that come with brain injuries. Through addressing the emotional impact, providing coping skills, and offering family advice, patients and their loved ones can navigate the emotional terrain of the recovery process with greater awareness. People can successfully manage the emotional challenges with assistance, knowledge, and communication, which will ultimately contribute to a more comprehensive and complete rehabilitation process.

CHAPTER 8

Long-Term Management and
Prevention Strategies

This chapter would focus on the ongoing management of head injury patients, including long-term medical follow-up, potential complications, and strategies to prevent future head injuries. It might also touch on lifestyle adjustments and safety measures.

Recuperation from a brain injury is a process that goes far beyond the initial phases. The important topic of long-term care and preventative measures for people with head injuries is covered in detail in Chapter 8. Head injury patients face many challenges during the post-injury phase of their lives. This chapter offers a comprehensive guide to ensuring their well-being and quality of life, from adopting lifestyle adjustments and addressing potential complications to implementing safety measures and continuing medical follow-up.

Ongoing Medical Monitoring:

The first step in long-term care is scheduling routine follow-up visits with a doctor to assess the patient's condition and handle any changing needs. Healthcare providers, such as neurologists and rehabilitation specialists, are essential in evaluating mental and physical functioning, monitoring possible problems, and modifying treatment regimens as necessary.

Managing Possible Difficulties:

Over time, a variety of potential consequences resulting from head injuries may surface. Chapter 8 lists a few of these issues, including:

Syndrome of Post-Concussion: Long after the initial injury, some people continue to have symptoms like headaches, dizziness, and cognitive impairments. The efficient management of these symptoms can be aided by a multidisciplinary approach combining psychologists, therapists, and medical practitioners.

2. Seizures and Epilepsy: Head trauma can result in seizures, particularly in cases of moderate to severe trauma. Seizures must be prevented and controlled with careful

observation and adequate management, which frequently includes antiepileptic drugs.

3. Mental and Cognitive Difficulties: A person may experience persistent or progressive behavioral changes, mood swings, and cognitive deficiencies over time. Support groups, counseling, and cognitive rehabilitation can help with managing these issues.

Modifications to Lifestyle:

To maintain the best possible quality of life, head injury patients and their families frequently need to undertake the following lifestyle changes:

1. Nutritious Diet and Exercise: Regular exercise and a balanced diet promote general health and may help with both physical and mental healing. Personalized advice can be obtained by speaking with a nutritionist or healthcare expert.

2. Sufficient Rest: Good sleep is essential for recuperation and cognitive function. Optimal recovery is facilitated by establishing a good sleep habit and resolving sleep problems.

3. Stress Management: Using relaxation methods and stress management strategies helps lessen the effects of psychological issues that may surface following a head injury.

Prevention and Safety Measures:

A crucial part of long-term care is preventing more brain injuries. This chapter highlights a number of preventative techniques:

1. Protective gear and helmets: The risk of head injuries is greatly decreased when wearing the proper

helmets and protective gear, whether playing sports, riding, or just relaxing.

2. Fall Prevention: It is imperative to take steps to prevent falls in older adults, such as eliminating trip hazards and making sure areas are well-lit.

3. Car Safety and Seat Belts: In order to reduce the risk of brain injuries in auto accidents, it is essential to wear seat belts and install car seats correctly.

4. Avoiding Risky Behaviors: Preventing injuries requires educating people about the possible dangers of

engaging in risky behaviors like drinking alcohol and acting carelessly.

Education-Related Initiatives:

Knowledge on head injury prevention and management is essential for head injury patients, their families, and the larger community. Campaigns for awareness, workshops, and educational programs can all be very effective in boosting security and lowering the number of head injuries.

Rendering:

The significance of long-term care and preventative measures for people with head injuries is emphasized in Chapter 8. This section provides a thorough road map for enhancing the wellbeing and quality of life of patients with brain injuries, covering everything from ongoing medical monitoring and handling possible problems to accepting lifestyle changes and putting safety precautions in place. It gives readers the knowledge and skills necessary to successfully negotiate the opportunities and difficulties of the post-injury phase by highlighting the importance of preventive care and continuing care, which promotes a comprehensive approach to resilience and recovery.